Dad's Building a Great Physique

A Step by Step Blueprint to Transforming Your Dadbod Once and For All

Introduction

Congratulations on purchasing this book! In doing so, you've taken the first step towards building the physique you've always wanted but didn't quite know how to get started. I became a dad to a beautiful little girl in November of 2018 and what a rollercoaster ride it's been! I want to be her hero. I want her to look at me and know that I'm her protector and I'll never let anything happen to her.

I can only assume that by purchasing this book, you would like your kids to see you in the same light. I can promise that if you take the concepts within this book and apply them with full force, there's absolutely no reason you can't take your physique to a whole new level and do just that.

I've spent my whole life learning the lessons I've written down on the following pages and used them to become a Pro Men's Physique Athlete and a Fitness Coach helping dads all around the world lose stubborn fat and build muscle. Now it's your turn.

By the time you're done reading, you'll have all the information you need to succeed in losing the stubborn belly fat and building rock-hard muscle in its place. All you'll need to do is take action!

And I know you will. See you on the other side.

Table of Contents

Chapter 1: Why Build a Physique?

When I was a kid, I always looked up to my dad. He was a big, strong, fit, and charming guy. We would shoot hoops in the driveway, play catch in the yard, go sledding at the park down the street, you name it. He was my first best friend and more importantly, my role model.

At first I thought that's how all dads must be. Big, strong, active, happy, and generally fun to be around. It wasn't until I started meeting my friends' dads that it all clicked.

My dad *wasn't* like most of the other dads.

From what I could see, most dads weren't big (at least not in the way I'd ever want to be). Most dads weren't active with their kids like mine was with me. They always seemed so grumpy, just sitting around watching TV. To the point that anytime my friends and I would get together, we'd all agree to just meet up at MY house!

My dad was always the life of the party too. He was so filled with energy, you could catch him doing push-ups in between commercial breaks when my family was watching TV. Since I wanted to be just like him, I'd plop down and knock out some push-ups too. I'd flex my biceps in pictures when he would flex his and drink protein shakes before bed with him (even though I'm pretty sure they were just milk with some ground up ice).

Hey, my dad was fit and charismatic, but he was also a cheap ass with the protein!

I always looked up to him and couldn't wait to grow up and become a man, so I could look just like him.

A few years later, when I was about 12 years old, that desire was fueled by an incident at the private pool my family belonged to. I was playing Knock Out in my swim trunks with my friends, when the girl I liked, Kimberly, approached me.

I started getting nervous.

Was she impressed that I won the last game? Would she want me to buy her something from the concession stand? Did I have any money on me if that was the case?

All these thoughts were flying through my head when her mouth opened, and she asked me point blank...

"Why are you so scrawny?"

I couldn't believe it. What the fuck kind of question is that? I just stood there, basketball in my hands, slowly starting to hold it in front of my stomach to cover up my pathetic ribs.

My first thought was, "Dad, you motherfucker, I knew you were hoarding all the protein!" After a few seconds (but what seemed like forever) I responded that I was going to be joining a weight lifting class soon and that should help put some muscle on me.

Of course, I was full of shit.

A few hours later, after my mom had picked me up and dropped me off at home, I scoured the house trying to find my dad. When I found him mowing the lawn out back, I asked him when the next time he was planning on hitting the gym.

"I just got back." He responded.

"Are you going back tomorrow?" I asked.

"Yeah but what's this all about?" He inquired.

"Can I go with you?" I asked as if my life depended on it.

Knowing that he couldn't bring any guests to his gym without paying a fee (again, cheap ass), he told me that there were some 15 lb dumbbells in the basement and that I should go down there every night after dinner and knock out 100 push-ups, 100 sit-ups, and 100 bicep curls.

Who could wait until after dinner? I all but sprinted downstairs to blow the dust off those rickety old dumbbells and got to work.

This went on for about 2 weeks. Every night I would ask my mom as she was serving dinner, "Is this healthy?" Automatically she would respond with, "Yes, spaghetti is healthy." or "Of course KFC is healthy. It's chicken!" I would then clear my plate, run downstairs, and get started on my routine.

By this time, 100 push-ups were nothing. I would be down in the basement for damn near an hour knocking out my work out until that one fateful day, I heard my dad call my name from up in the kitchen. When I went up there, he asked me how my workouts had been going. I told him I thought my muscles were starting to grow, but I wasn't positive.

That's when it happened. He asked me, "How would you like me to take you to the gym tomorrow to show you some more stuff?"

Was this really happening?

Kimberly's going to be so impressed when she sees me at the pool next summer. I bet I'll be frickin' huge!

"Sounds good! Let's celebrate by having a protein shake!" I said as I eagle-eyed him, making sure he didn't short me.

The next day, as we walked into the gym, it was like nothing I had ever seen before. Guys with huge muscles talking to girls with big butts. Did my mom know that my dad was coming here? Was this paradise?

I followed my dad around like a lost puppy as he took me through some of the easier exercises that he thought a 12-year-old could handle. About 45 minutes later, after our final set of tricep rope pushdowns, he asked if I was ready to go home and eat.

"We're coming back tomorrow, right?" I asked.

"Sure." He replied.

Going to the gym with my dad was easily my favorite part of growing up. We got to talk about how nuts my mom and sister were, talk about girls, and I got to ask him questions I normally would have never felt comfortable asking. This was our way of bonding for years and has always been a tradition I've wanted to carry on with my kids when they got to that age.

I'm happy to say that about 20 years later, my old man is still getting it done. And I'll be damned if he's getting to the gym after delivering mail for 12 hours a day at 55 years old and I'm not because of some bull shit excuse!

Since being that 12-year-old boy, my passion (obsession) with building a great physique has only amplified. Do I want to be the scrawny husband at the lake? Or the ripped husband my wife can be proud of? Do I want to be the active dad for my kids? Or do I want to be the couch potato?

These are the reasons I get to the gym consistently. Now you just must ask yourself, why will you?

Chapter 2: Why Motivation Is Bullshit and What You'll Actually Need Instead

It's a crazy phenomenon I've noticed year after year. The day after a Rocky marathon is played on TV, the number of middle-aged guys working out at my local gym damn near triples. The day after that, a few stragglers (the ones with the Eye of the Tiger, I imagine) come back to get another session in. By day three, it's back to just the regulars.

Why is this? (Hint: It's not because they're at home chasing chickens or running stairs like Balboa.)

It's because of the temporary high you experience with motivation. Motivation gets your blood pumping, your adrenaline flowing, and you feel like you can do just about anything. The problem with motivation is that it's temporary. It's like a sugar rush where you feel on top of the world for a while, only to come crashing down an hour or so later.

Whether it's catching yourself getting out of breath from doing basic activities like walking up a few flights of stairs, or no longer being able to fit into the jeans you've been wearing for the last five years because "they mysteriously shrunk," these things are likely to give you that little spark of motivation.

Just enough motivation to say to yourself, "That's it! I'm cutting out all the junk food and carbs. Only meat and vegetables for me until I get back to where I want to be!" Nonetheless a day or two later, somebody brings pizza to the office or your kids don't finish their macaroni and cheese at dinner.

Suddenly, that little voice in your head starts saying, "Hey man. You've been strict for a few days now. And you're already down a few pounds! You might as well indulge now and just get back on track tomorrow."

However, "tomorrow" doesn't come until a few weeks later, when you're on the couch eating Cheetos and see Gerard Butler's abs in 300. Then, what do you know? The cycle repeats and you're motivated again.

You see, that tiny spark of motivation is great but it's just not enough to make lasting, life-altering changes. So, what do you need instead? Simple.

Commitment.

If you're going to make any lasting changes, you'll need to fully understand that the process is going to SUCK and embrace it. It's going to suck a lot at first, suck a little less a month down the road, and a few months after that, it'll only suck a little bit. Before you know it, you'll have started seeing REAL results, and it won't suck at all anymore.

You'll be addicted.

Don't have the willpower to fight through those first few months by yourself? Find somebody that will hold you accountable.

I already know what you're thinking...

"That's not necessary, if I really buckle down and commit I know I can do it."

It's not your fault for thinking that way, it's human nature. It's also completely and utterly false. How many years have you had to do it? How many times have you tried and failed by yourself? What'll make this time any different? Nothing will.

Instead, pick one of the following options.

Option 1: Find a workout buddy that's ALREADY committed to hitting the gym.

This shouldn't be a friend or significant other that's "trying to get back into it" just like you are. They're in the same place you are! You wouldn't ask your drunk friend to drive you home because you've had too many beers. So why would you ask somebody who has never been consistent to hold you accountable?

Instead, you'll need to find somebody that has been consistent for YEARS and tell them to MAKE YOU GO. Hell, give them some money and tell them it's theirs at the end of the month if you fail to show up even once.

Option 2: Hire a coach.

Hiring a coach is a great way to get the added accountability. Not only will they help you see results quicker by dialing in on your training and nutrition, technology is to the point that they can see the moment you start slacking and call you out on it.

Not to mention, by investing in a coach, you now have what's known as "skin in the game." As a fitness coach myself, I've seen a direct correlation between those that I offer to help for free, and those who I charge. Those that I try to help for free quickly bypass my advice and look for "another secret way" to hopefully see immediate results. And why wouldn't they? They won't be out ANYTHING if they don't stick to my program.

Those who do have skin in the game listen to what I have to say, put it into action, and see great results as a biproduct.

There are plenty of coaches out there that you can get help from, but I recommend doing your homework first. You don't want a coach that doesn't look the way you want to look (aka practice what they preach). You don't want a coach that takes steroids because what has worked for them certainly won't work for you. You know what? Save yourself the time and effort right now and just shoot me an email at joel@joelstaleyfitness.com.

If I'm not available to coach you or we're just not a good fit, I have a great network of other coaches that I can recommend for you.

Option 3: Become part of a like-minded community.

Although not quite as effective as the first two options, becoming a part of a like-minded community can help drive adherence. Facebook groups or small training gyms are a great place to form or join these communities.

You can join our Private Facebook Group 'Dads Who Lift' at: https://www.facebook.com/groups/Dads.Who.Lift/

Although motivation can be a great way to get off the couch, you'll be hard pressed to ride that short wave all the way to the shore that is your dream physique. Instead, realize that it will suck for a while until you get some momentum going, and choose one or more of those three options to help increase accountability that will keep you in it for the long run.

Chapter 3: How to Set Up Your

Workout Routine

Have you ever watched The Biggest Loser or one of those other weight loss shows and thought to yourself..."Those poor bastards!"

Running up flights of stadium stairs, puking over the railing of the elliptical, flipping tires until their whole body cramps up and they break down in tears. If that's what it takes to build a great physique, count me out!

Yet, that's the message they're broadcasting and that's what a lot of people take to be the truth. So, if that's the truth, why do over 90% of those contestants gain back the weight plus more? And why don't the guys with the best physiques in the world train anything like that? For a couple reasons.

The contestants on those shows focus on an insane, unsustainable amount of cardio, for one. When the show's over, and their bodies have adapted to only eating 1200 calories and rowing for 7 hours every day, as soon as they slow down, the weight comes right back.

Because of the high demand they put on their bodies, their metabolism slows way down making it hard to keep the weight off. And to boot, after the show's over, they're sent back home not knowing anything about how to program their diet or training! Kind of messed up when you think about it, but hey, I guess that's reality TV for ya.

So, what's the right answer if you want to build muscle and lose fat permanently? Four words.

Resistance Training and Diet.

Resistance training (aka weightlifting) enables you to build muscle. Muscle is what's known as an *"expensive tissue"* meaning it takes a lot of calories to sustain it. Simply put, the more muscle you build, the more calories you burn.

Think of cardio like playing defense and resistance training like playing offense. You have a cheat meal and your first thought is to do cardio to "offset" those extra calories, (defense). Or you focus on lifting weights so those added calories go towards building muscle, muscle that will BURN more calories, (offense)!

The more cardio you do, the more your metabolism slows down, and the more weightlifting you do, the more your metabolism revs up. Does that mean that if you go to the gym and start popping off some bicep curls, suddenly you can eat whatever you want? Of course not.

When resistance training, if your goal is to build lean muscle and burn stubborn body fat, you should focus on what are known as Compound Lifts.

So, what's a compound lift?

Lifts can be classified as either:

Compound (which involve more than one muscle group) or **Isolation** (which isolate only one muscle group at a time).

For Example:

Bicep curls only target the biceps. They would be classified as an isolation lift.

Deadlifts target the hamstrings, quads, butt, thighs, lower back, and traps. They would be classified as a compound lift.

Other compound lifts include:

Squats (complete lower body and core)

Bench Press (chest, triceps, and shoulders)

Overhead Press (shoulders, triceps, and core)

Bent Over Barbell Rows (lats, rhomboids, traps, rear deltoids, and biceps)

Pull Ups (lats, biceps, traps, triceps, and upper chest)

Dips (triceps, chest, and deltoids)

-

Bicep curls and other isolation exercises certainly have their place but if your overall goal is to lose fat, compound lifts are going to burn the most calories.

If your goal is to build muscle, compound lifts will target the most amount of muscle being used and therefore build the most muscle. (Remember the offense we talked about?)

If your goal is to *lose fat and build muscle*, you definitely can't afford to skip out on compound lifts.

-

Now that we got that out of the way, you'll have to **decide how many days each week you can commit to hitting the gym**.

If you're starting from scratch, LESS IS MORE! You don't want to start off going six days a week, get burnt out, and throw in the towel altogether.

Plus, it won't do you any good! If your body isn't used to lifting and you suddenly start going six days a week, your body will focus on RECOVERING instead of focusing on BUILDING MUSCLE which is what we want it to do.

So realistically, how many times a week (every week) can you commit to going to the gym for the next six months?

2 or 3 Days a Week

If you can only go to the gym two or three days a week, you'll want to focus on Full Body Workouts. Full Body Workouts do just as they say, train your whole body.

The benefits of Full Body Workouts are that you can still hit every muscle group multiple times each week. This will force them to grow and be much more effective than just hitting them only once a week.

Below are some sample routines for training both two and three days a week.

-

2 Day Split

-

Monday

Barbell Bench Press (4 sets of 10)

Bent Over Rows (4 sets of 10)

Overhead Press (4 sets of 10)

Squats (4 sets of 10)

Plank (4 sets of 30 seconds)

Thursday

Incline Bench Press (5 sets of 8)

Pull Ups or Lat Pulldown (5 sets of 8)

Dumbbell Shoulder Press (5 sets of 8)

Lunges (5 sets of 8)

Crunches (5 sets of 20)

-

3 Day Split

\-

Monday

Barbell Bench Press (4 sets of 10)

Bent Over Rows (4 sets of 10)

Overhead Press (4 sets of 10)

Squats (4 sets of 10)

Plank (4 sets of 10)

Wednesday

Incline Bench Press (5 sets of 8)

Pull Ups or Lat Pulldown (5 sets of 8)

Dumbbell Shoulder Press (5 sets of 8)

Lunges (5 sets of 8)

Crunches (5 sets of 20)

Friday

Deadlifts (4 sets of 12)

Dumbbell Bench Press (4 sets of 12)

Military Press (4 sets of 12)

Front Squats (4 sets of 12)

Hanging Leg Raises (4 sets of 12)

\-

If you're doing Full Body Workouts, you'll want to leave at least 36-48 hours in between training sessions. This will allow your muscles to recover, rebuild, and come back bigger and stronger. Remember, muscles are torn apart in the gym and grow during rest and recovery. If you never give them a chance to recover, you may end up doing more harm than good.

-

4 Days a Week

If you decide you want to train four times a week, I highly recommend doing what's known as an Upper/Lower Split. This means you'll alternate between working the muscles in your upper body (shoulders, arms, chest, and back) and working the muscles in your lower body (butt, quads, hamstrings, thighs, and calves). It may look something like this.

-

Monday – Upper Body I

Overhead Press (4 sets of 12)

Dumbbell Bench Press (4 sets of 12)

Barbell Row (4 sets of 12)

DB Curls (4 sets of 12)

Tricep Dips (4 sets of 12)

Tuesday – Lower Body I

Squats (4 sets of 12)

Leg Extensions (4 sets of 12)

Romanian Deadlifts (4 sets of 12)

Thigh Abductor (4 sets of 12)

Seated Calf Raises (4 sets of 12)

Thursday – Upper Body II

Dumbbell Shoulder Press (5 sets of 8)

Incline Bench Press (5 sets of 8)

Single Arm Row (5 sets of 8)

Hammer Curls (5 sets of 8)

Tricep Kickbacks (5 sets of 8)

Friday – Lower Body II

Front Squats (5 sets of 8)

Lunges (5 sets of 8)

Seated Leg Curls (5 sets of 8)

Thigh Adductor (5 sets of 8)

Smith Machine Calf Raises (4 sets of 15)

-

While doing an Upper/Lower Split, you'll just want to make sure that you aren't training the same muscle groups two days in a row (example: Monday: Upper Body I and Tuesday: Upper Body II).

-

5 Days a Week.

Training five times a week is a little less black and white. There are several ways you can go about it, but you'll want to make sure you're still hitting each muscle group at least twice. You'll want to stay away from the Mon: Chest, Tuesday: Back, Wednesday: Arms, etc. type of routine because this will only allow you to train everything once each week which is suboptimal.

One thing you can do is to have an Upper/Lower Split with one Full Body Workout added.

-

Monday – Upper Body I
Overhead Press (4 sets of 12)
Dumbbell Bench Press (4 sets of 12)
Barbell Row (4 sets of 12)
DB Curls (4 sets of 12)
Triceps Dips (4 sets of 12)

Tuesday – Lower Body I

Squats (4 sets of 12)

Leg Extensions (4 sets of 12)

Romanian Deadlifts (4 sets of 12)

Thigh Abductor (4 sets of 12)

Seated Calf Raises (4 sets of 12)

Wednesday – Upper Body II

Dumbbell Shoulder Press (5 sets of 8)

Incline Bench Press (5 sets of 8)

Single Arm Row (5 sets of 8)

Hammer Curls (5 sets of 8)

Triceps Kickbacks (5 sets of 8)

Thursday – Lower Body II

Front Squats (5 sets of 8)

Lunges (5 sets of 8)

Seated Leg Curls (5 sets of 8)

Thigh Adductor (5 sets of 8)

Smith Machine Calf Raises (4 sets of 15)

Saturday – Full Body Workout

Deadlifts (4 sets of 12)

Dumbbell Bench Press (4 sets of 12)

Military Press (4 sets of 12)

Sumo Squats (4 sets of 12)

Hanging Leg Raises (4 sets of 12)

-

6 Days a Week.

Training six days a week is great for experienced lifters and something you'll want to possibly build up to someday, however it's not a great place to start from scratch. The process of building muscle is caused by continually adding volume over time and if you start with this much volume, it'll be extremely difficult to keep progressing month after month.

Once you ARE ready, I'd highly recommend a Push/Pull/Legs Routine. This means you'll be working your upper body muscles responsible for pushing movements (shoulders, chest, and triceps) on one day, your upper body muscles responsible for pulling (back, biceps, and rear delts) on another day, and legs (butt, hamstrings, quads, thighs, and calves) on the other day. You'll then repeat this process throughout the week while taking one rest day, giving you six full days of training.

-

Push/Pull/Legs Routine

-

Monday – Push Workout I

Incline Barbell Bench Press (4 sets of 12)

Push-Ups (4 sets of 20)

Standing Dumbbell Press (4 sets of 12)

Lateral Raises (4 sets of 12)

Close Grip Bench (4 sets of 12)

Triceps Dips (4 sets of 12)

Tuesday – Pull Workout I

Barbell Rows (4 sets of 12)

Pull Ups (4 sets of 10)

Barbell Curls (4 sets of 12)

Hammer Curls (4 sets of 12)

Rear Delt Flyes (4 sets of 12)

Rope Face Pulls (4 sets of 12)

Wednesday – Leg Day I

Squats (4 sets of 12)

Leg Extensions (4 sets of 12)

Romanian Deadlifts (4 sets of 12)

Thigh Abductor (4 sets of 12)

Seated Calf Raises (4 sets of 12)

Friday – Push Workout II

Barbell Bench Press (5 sets of 8)

Chest Flyes (4 sets of 15)

Military Press (5 sets of 8)

Upright Rows (5 sets of 10)

Triceps Rope Pushdowns (5 sets of 10)

Tricep Kickbacks (4 sets of 12)

Saturday – Pull Workout II

Single Arm Rows (5 sets of 8)

Lat Pulldowns (5 sets of 8)

Dumbbell Curls (5 sets of 8)

Reverse Curls (5 sets of 8)

Rear Delt Cable Flyes (5 sets of 8)

Rope Face Pulls (4 sets of 20)

Sunday – Leg Day II

Front Squats (5 sets of 8)

Lunges (5 sets of 8)

Seated Leg Curls (5 sets of 8)

Thigh Adductor (5 sets of 8)

Smith Machine Calf Raises (4 sets of 15)

-

Although the Push/Pull/Legs Split is the most common, there's nothing to say that you couldn't do an Upper/Lower Split instead, working both muscle groups three times each week.

You'll notice I didn't make options for training only once a week, nor training seven days a week. Training only once a week, while better than nothing, will be tough to build a physique with such a small amount of volume. As far as training seven days a week goes, remember that your muscles will need time to recover and you'll be much better off giving yourself at least one or two days off to rest up each week.

Chapter 4: Training – Common Weightlifting Mistakes

There's a lot of misinformation when it comes to lifting weights. The bottom line is, if you work hard enough for long enough, and your diet is decent, you'll make progress. With that being said, if you're looking to build and sculpt your physique in the quickest and most effective way possible, you'll want to avoid some of these common mistakes. To understand most of these, you'll first have to understand what Progressive Overload is.

Progressive Overload is the act of steadily increasing your *training volume* over time.

Training Volume is the total amount of weight lifted for a specific exercise.

For example:

If you bench press 200 lbs. for 4 sets of 10 reps, your **volume** would be **8,000 lbs.** (or 200 lbs. x 4 x 10).

In order to **progress** the next week, you'd have to make sure to **increase volume**.

You could do this one of three ways:

Increasing the amount of weight lifted: **210 lbs.** x 4 x 10 = 8,400 lbs. - (a 400 lb. increase in volume)

Increasing the amount of reps performed: 200 lbs. x 4 x **12** = 9,600 lbs. - (a 1,600 lb. increase in volume)

Increasing the amount of sets performed: 200 lbs. x **5** x 10 = 10,000 lbs. - (a 2,000 lb. increase in volume)

Now that you understand Progressive Overload and its importance to building muscle, let's get into some of the common mistakes.

1) Training to Failure on Every Set

It's extremely common for guys in the gym trying to build muscle to lift until failure on every set. What this means is that they perform every set of every workout until the point they cannot do even one more rep. The problem with this is that training to failure on the first few sets impairs the amount of volume you can lift in the following sets.

Let's bring it back to our bench press example from above.

If you can bench 200 lbs. for 10 reps and fail before 11, your sets may go something like this.

First Set: 200 lbs. for 10 reps.

Second Set: 200 lbs. and fail at 9 reps.

Third Set: 200 lbs. and fail at 7 reps.

Fourth Set: 200 lbs. and fail at 5 reps.

Total Volume: 6,200 lbs.

-

Now let's say you cut it a few reps short of failure and left some "reps in the tank" for the first few sets. Then, took the *last set* to failure since it wouldn't impact any subsequent sets.

-

First Set: 200 lbs. and stop at 8 reps.

Second Set: 200 lbs. and stop at 8 reps.

Third Set: 200 lbs. and stop at 8 reps.

Fourth Set: 200 lbs. and fail at 10 reps.

Total Volume: 6,800 lbs.

-

As you can imagine, a 600 lb. difference in volume would add up substantially over time. Assuming you do six workouts a day for four days a week with this type of difference, you'd be missing out on 432,000 lbs. of volume in just one month!

Don't think that not going to failure on every set will mean that you're not getting a good workout. Volume is what's important here.

On the other hand, you also can't forget about *intensity*. If you're leaving 3, 4, 5 reps in the tank on every set, chances are you're not going in with the intensity needed to build muscle. You'll want to find a happy medium between maximizing volume and intensity to get the results you're looking for. Stopping 1 or 2 reps short is usually a great way to get the best of both worlds.

-

2) Not Tracking Your Workouts

Like I mentioned in the introduction to this chapter, Progressive Overload is the most important aspect of building muscle.

If you're not tracking your workouts, you're not tracking your volume. If you're not tracking your volume, you can't possibly know if you're progressing week to week.

Whether you go as far as bringing a notebook to the gym, or just use an app on your phone, you'll want to make sure you're tracking the amount of weight, reps, and sets for each exercise of every single workout. This way, you can compare them with the previous weeks to make sure you're continuing to progress. Some apps you could download to track volume include HeavySet (iOS), Strong (iOS, Android), and Fitbod (iOS).

-

3) Switching Up Your Workouts Every Week

You shouldn't switch up your workouts every week for the same reason you need to track. At the risk of sounding like a broken record, Progressive Overload.

If I squat 300 lbs. for 4 sets of 10 this week, that's a training volume of 12,000 lbs.

If I do lunges next week with 80 lb. dumbbells for 4 sets of 10, that's a training volume of 3,200 lbs.

Did I progress?

Who the hell knows!? They're completely different exercises!

On the other hand, if I squat 300 lbs. for 4 sets of 10 this week, (12,000 lbs.) and squat 310 lbs. for 4 sets of 10 next week (12,400 lbs.), did I progress?

Pretty easy to see that I did by 400 lbs.

That's why switching up your workouts every week is a huge mistake. It makes it damn near impossible to see whether you've actually progressed or not. Instead, stick to the same program for AT LEAST three to six weeks so you can consistently and reliably track your progress.

-

4) Not Doing Enough Compound Lifts

Like I mentioned in Chapter 3, if you're looking to get stronger, build muscle, and burn fat, compound lifts are going to be your best friend.

As a reminder, lifts can be classified as either:

Compound - which involve more than one muscle group.

Or

Isolation - which isolate only one muscle group at a time.

-

Examples of <u>Compound Lifts</u> include:

Deadlifts (hamstrings, quads, butt, thighs, lower back, and traps)

Squats (complete lower body and core)

Bench Press (chest, triceps, and shoulders)

Overhead Press (shoulders, triceps, and core)

Bent Over Barbell Rows (lats, rhomboids, traps, rear deltoids, and biceps)

Pull Ups (lats, biceps, traps, triceps, and upper chest)

Dips (triceps, chest, and deltoids)

-

Examples of <u>Isolation Lifts</u> include:

Leg Extensions (Quads)

Leg Curls (Hamstrings)

Bicep Curls (Biceps)

Tricep Kickbacks (Triceps)

Lateral Raise (Shoulders)

Dumbbell Flyes (Chest)

Calf Raises (Calves)

Straight Arm Pulldowns (Back)

-

I wouldn't advise cutting out Isolation Lifts altogether by any means, but you'll definitely want to prioritize Compound Lifts. Think of Compound Lifts as the John Deer lawn mower and Isolation Exercises as the weedwhacker. Sure, a weedwhacker is great for making the final touches, but you'd have an extremely hard time keeping your lawn in check without the lawn mower.

-

5) Not Using Full Range of Motion

If you've been in the gym even once, you've probably seen somebody doing pull ups without even breaking 90 degrees, doing curls within a 6-inch span, or squatting without really even bending their knees at all.

Usually these guys are what is known as "Ego Lifters" using a weight that's way more than they should be attempting to lift.

Simply put, someone squatting 200 lbs. with good form and full range of motion (ROM) will be way better off than someone else squatting 600 lbs. and barely breaking at the knee.

If the amount of weight you're lifting keeps going up, but the range of motion that you're using keeps getting shorter, this is not considered progress and won't help you build that awesome physique you're looking to build.

Start with a weight that you're confident with, practice using full ROM, and gradually increase the weight as you go.

-

6) Going in the Gym Without a Plan

This one's rather self-explanatory and goes hand in hand with not tracking and/or switching up your workouts every week. If you go into the gym without a plan (although better than not going into the gym at all) it will be impossible to track your progress from your previous workouts.

If you have a plan but forgot it at home or are unable to access it for some reason, it's not going to make or break your progress if you go to the gym once or twice and do a workout off the cuff. Having said that, if you're consistently going to the gym and just doing whatever exercises come to mind at that exact moment, you'll have a much harder time building your physique than somebody who's following a strict regimen and focusing on Progressive Overload.

-

7) Never Switching Up Your Workouts

Although switching up your workouts too often isn't beneficial because it doesn't give your body enough time to adapt, you also want to be mindful that you don't get stuck doing the same routine for too long.

You wouldn't keep working at the same job if you got paid less and less each month, would you?

Well that's exactly what happens when you stay in the same routine for too long. After a while, the muscle adaptation benefits become less and less effective until finally, you stop seeing results altogether.

This is known as the *Law of Diminishing Returns.*

Although everybody's different, usually 8 weeks is the longest I'd recommend sticking to the same workouts before making some changes.

-

8) Staying Within the Same Rep Range for Too Long

The Law of Diminishing Returns doesn't only apply to workouts, but also the amount of reps you perform.

Generally speaking, you should stay within:

-

1-5 reps if your goal is STRENGTH

8-12 reps if your goal is HYPERTROPHY (aka building muscle)

And **15+ reps** if your goal is ENDURANCE

Although these give a pretty good indicator of where your focus should be depending on your specific goal, the longer you stay in one of these ranges, the less benefit you'll receive. That's why, even if your goal is to build muscle (which it should be if you're reading this book), you won't want to stay in the 8-12 rep range forever.

An example of how you might structure your periodization may look something like this:

January: 8-12 rep range

February: 4-6 rep range

March: 12-15 rep range

April: 1-5 rep range

May: 15-20 rep range

(Repeat)

That's not to say you can't work within multiple rep ranges at once. A lot of programs will have you hit each muscle group twice a week, one focusing on building muscle (8-12) and one focusing on gaining strength (1-5).

9) Not Spending Enough Time Under Tension

Time Under Tension is calculated by how long your muscle stays under tension. Basically, it's how long it takes you to complete one full rep of any given exercise.

Take the bicep curl for example.

The dumbbell starts down by your thigh and you contract your bicep to bring the dumbbell up by your shoulder. (You just did the motion didn't you?)

This is what's known as a CONCENTRIC contraction (aka squeezing your muscle).

The act of lowering the dumbbell back down towards your thigh is what's known as an ECCENTRIC contraction (aka stretching the muscle).

Time Under Tension refers to how long it takes you to go through both the concentric contraction and the eccentric contraction, aka doing one full bicep curl.

Say it takes you **one second to bring the dumbbell up,** and **three seconds to bring the dumbbell down**.

This would put your TUT at four seconds for that one rep.

Now say you did ten reps just like this. That would put your TUT at 40 seconds.

Since **most of the muscle building benefits comes from the eccentric** (or lowering) of the weight, you don't want to rush it.

If you were to do bicep curls and the full rep only took you two seconds (one second up and one second down), you'd be much better off slowing down and trying to stretch your TUT out to four seconds (one second up and three seconds down).

Long story short, take your time and control the weight that you're lifting. Don't use momentum and rush your way through it or you'll have a tougher time building muscle and put yourself at an increased risk of injury.

Chapter 5 – How to Structure Your Diet

Sometimes it seems impossible to eat clean. The kids leave half their dinner to be thrown away, so you have to help them out. Your wife is on you to take her to that new pasta place. Plus, who can control those late-night cravings that seem to pop up every night around 9 pm?

How could any dad build a physique in these types of conditions!?

It's not quite as complicated as you may have been led to believe.

What took me forever to figure out, and 90% of guys still don't understand, is that you don't need to eat perfectly to build the physique you've always wanted. Too good to be true, right?

Wrong!

If you're anything like I used to be, you probably think you need to eat only "clean foods" (chicken, salads, cans of tuna, egg whites, etc.) to build a great physique.

NOPE!

In fact, weight loss comes down to one thing.

Calories.

The fundamental truth is that if you burn more calories than you eat, you'll LOSE weight.

On the other hand, if you eat more calories than you burn, you'll GAIN weight!

-

The fact is, somebody who eats 1,500 calories of pizza a day will lose more weight than somebody who eats 1,600 calories worth of salad!

Crazy, right!?

Obviously, the salad would be a *healthier* option, but we're talking about gaining and losing weight, not optimizing our health quite yet.

So how many calories should you eat?

Here's a quick rule of thumb.

-

If you want to BUILD MUSCLE: Eat (Your Weight x 20 calories per day)

If you want to MAINTAIN: Eat (Your Weight x 15 calories per day)

If you want to LOSE FAT: Eat (Your Weight x 10 calories per day)

-

Not sure how to track your calories? It really couldn't be any easier.

Downloadable apps such as **MyFitnessPal** make for extremely easy calorie counting. All you have to do is plug in the foods you eat and the app will deduct that number of calories from your daily goal as you go.

-

Unfortunately, that's only a piece of the puzzle. A major piece, but only a piece nonetheless.

The next major piece, is…

PROTEIN.

As we just discussed, if you eat less calories than you burn, you will lose WEIGHT.

However, if you don't get enough protein, some of that weight loss will come from MUSCLE.

That's NOT what we want!

-

Luckily for us, when we **lift weights** and **eat enough protein**, most (or all) of that weight will come from unwanted FAT.

That means you'll be able to lose the belly and still be able to retain or even keep building muscle.

-

As for how much protein, you should <u>aim to get around one gram per pound of body weight</u> each day.

-

If you weigh 110 lbs., eat 110 grams of protein each day.

If you weigh 150 lbs., eat 150 grams of protein each day.

If you weigh 220 lbs., eat 220 grams of protein each day.

(220 grams should be about the most you'll need even if you weigh much more than this).

-

For Reference:

8 oz Steak - 57 grams of protein

8 oz Beef - 48 grams of protein

8 oz Chicken - 44 grams of protein

2 Scoops Whey Protein Powder - 50 grams of protein

-

Don't want to track your protein? That's okay.

If you're the type of person that doesn't like to track, the next best thing you can do is this:

Try to have at least one item that contains a lot of protein with each meal.

Also, consider incorporating a protein shake post workout.

-

Foods that contain a lot of protein include:

- Chicken

- Pork
- Beef
- Fish
- Turkey
- Eggs
- Egg Whites
- Beans
- Protein Bars
- Whey protein

…and much more.

That means you'll be able to lose the belly and still be able to retain or even keep building muscle.

-

Key Takeaways so far:

1) To lose weight, you must be in a caloric deficit.

2) To make sure that weight comes from FAT, you have to eat enough protein and also lift weights.

Next up…

CARBS.

Carbs are a great source of energy and can play a huge role in building muscle.

Out of the three macronutrients (Protein, Carbs, and Fat) the only one that we can live completely without is carbohydrates making it nonessential.

There are three different types of carbs:

Simple Starchy Carbohydrates

- Fructose - Found in fruit
- Glucose - Table sugar
- Lactose - Found in milk and dairy products

Complex Starchy Carbohydrates

- Rice
- Potatoes
- Pasta
- Bread

and **Complex Fibrous Carbohydrates**

- Vegetables

If your main goal is to **BUILD MUSCLE**, carbs should make up **between 40% - 60% of your diet**.

If your main goal is to **LOSE FAT**, you should stick **between 5% - 40% of your calories coming from carbs**.

You can build a lean muscular physique with or without carbs, but carbs will make the muscle building process much easier. There's no secret answer when it comes to carb consumption (although I can confidently say that you're better off limiting the sweets). At the end of the day, you have to find what works best for your lifestyle!

And finally, the last of the macronutrients...

FATS.

The myth that all fats are bad for you couldn't be further from the truth. Assuming that they are bad may just be one of the BIGGEST dietary mistakes people make. In fact, fats play a vital role in hormone production such as testosterone and help dramatically with both burning fat and building muscle. Just like protein, fat is essential and must be consumed to live.

Here are some of the fats you'll want to make sure you're getting enough of, and some you'll want to leave off your plate.

-

Good Fats

-

Monounsaturated Fats

- Avocados
- Canola, Sesame, and Olive Oils
- Peanut Butter/Nuts

- Olives

-

Polyunsaturated Fats

- Fatty Fish
- Flax Seeds
- Tofu
- Walnuts
- Soy Milk

-

Saturated fats

- Steak
- Beef
- Chicken Skin
- Butter

-

Bad Fats

-

- Trans Fats
- Pastries
- Chips
- Snack Foods
- Fried Foods
- Margarine

-

Here's a good rule of thumb.

Nature doesn't make bad fats, only companies do. Stick to this way of thinking and you really can't go wrong.

Chapter 6: How to Eat What You Want, And Look How You Want (Yes, really!)

For my 2015 New Year's Resolution, I wanted to compete in my first Men's Physique Show. I bought a 1-page diet plan for $250 that had everything I had to eat, every day until the show.

Meal 1) Egg Whites and Oatmeal.

Meal 2) Chicken, Sweet Potato, and Asparagus.

Meal 3) Tilapia, Rice, and Broccoli.

Meal 4) Salmon, Sweet Potato, and an Apple.

Meal 5) Protein Shake.

I ate these meals every day for 12 weeks straight, refusing to venture outside of this meal plan whatsoever. At one point, my wife even dared me to eat a piece of popcorn while we were sitting on the couch watching movies one night. Since it wasn't on my little laminated sheet, I declined. I was irritable, tired, and lethargic, but determined to see out my 12 weeks.

When my show day did finally arrive, I remember hearing another competitor talking backstage about how he had been eating donuts, Chinese food, and Taco Bell leading up to the show. At first, I thought he was just full of shit.

The guy was ripped, there was no way! Like I said, I had always been under the impression that you had to "eat clean" to look like that. That's what I had to do!

I went home, smashed a bunch of the foods I'd been craving for the last three months, and started researching this "Flexible Dieting" technique. Turns out, the other competitor wasn't lying!

This is when I found out that you have to eat less calories than you burn to lose weight, and if you lift weights and get enough protein, that weight will come from fat. So, in a nutshell, as long as I was eating less calories than I burned and getting enough protein, I could have eaten something like this instead and gotten the SAME RESULTS.

-

Meal 1) Glazed Donut.

Meal 2) Chicken and Asparagus.

Meal 3) Tilapia, Rice, and Broccoli.

Meal 4) 2 Taco Bell Softshell Beef Tacos and a Diet Coke.

Meal 5) Protein Shake (and some popcorn).

-

This was a GAME CHANGER for me. I went from, "I'm definitely never going to compete again, I can't do this" to "Wow, I can eat the foods I love and still stay ripped all year!" Come to find out, this way of eating known as "Flexible Dieting" was also known as IIFYM (or If It Fits Your Macros).

If you recall, **macros (or macronutrients) are just another name for protein, carbs, and fat**.

There are FOUR calories in every gram of protein, FOUR calories in every gram of carbs, and NINE calories in every gram of fat.

(This will be important to remember soon).

In the next section, I'll teach you how to calculate your macros so that you can eat what you want AND look how you want.

-

How to Calculate Your Macros

There are four steps to calculating your macros:

Step 1. Figure Out How Many Calories You Should Be Consuming Each Day.

Step 2. Figure Out How Much Protein You Should Be Consuming Each Day.

Step 3. Calculate How Much Fat You Should Be Consuming Each Day.

Step 4. Calculate How Many Carbs You Should Be Consuming Each Day.

In all honesty, as long as you figure out the first two steps (which happen to be the easiest) you can still get away with eating what you want. Carbs and fats, in the grand scheme of things, aren't quite as important if your calories and protein needs are being taken care of. So, don't let the math scare you away thinking you can't do this. Okay, here we go...

-

Get your notepad ready!

-

Step 1. Figure Out How Many Calories You Should Be Consuming Each Day.

Remember my rule of thumb:

-

If you want to BUILD MUSCLE: Eat (Your Weight x 20 calories per day)

If you want to MAINTAIN: Eat (Your Weight x 15 calories per day)

If you want to LOSE FAT: Eat (Your Weight x 10 calories per day)

-

(or just google a calorie calculator and input your sex, weight, height, activity level, etc., which will be more accurate).

-

Example: Right now, I am 185 lbs. So, depending on my goal...

-

185 lbs. x 20 calories = 3,700 calories/ day to BUILD MUSCLE
185 lbs. x 15 calories = 2,775 calories/ day to MAINTAIN
185 lbs. x 10 calories = 1,850 calories/ day to LOSE FAT
(For this example, let's just say I'd like to maintain and use 2,775 calories).

-

Step 2. Figure Out How Much Protein You Should Be Consuming Each Day.

Take your bodyweight and aim to consume that many *grams* of protein each day.

Example: My current weight is 185 lbs. = 185 grams per day. Easy enough?

-

Step 3. Calculate How Much Fat You Should Be Consuming Each Day.

Fat should make up at least 20% of your total calories.

Take your total daily calories and multiple by 0.20 (which gives you 20%)

This will give you how many calories of fat you should consume each day.

Unfortunately, we're looking for grams.

Knowing that there are NINE calories in one gram of fat, take the number of calories in fat and divide by nine to get your # of grams.

Using my example, my daily calories are 2,775.

2,775 x 0.20 = 555 calories from fat is what I want to shoot for.

To get that in grams, divide it by nine.

555/9 = 61.6 grams

So let's say I will want to get around 62 grams of fat each day.

Confused yet? I thought so. Don't worry, I'll bail you out at the end.

-

Step 4. Calculate How Many Carbs You Should Be Consuming Each Day.

After protein and fat needs are met, all of your remaining calories can go towards carbs.

Since there are FOUR calories in a gram of protein, take your protein in grams and multiply by four to get calories in protein.

Using my example: 185 lbs. x 4 = 740 calories in protein.

We also figured out in step 3 that my fat calories are 555.

ADD YOUR PROTEIN CALORIES AND FAT CALORIES TOGETHER, THEN SUBTRACT FROM YOUR TOTAL DAILY CALORIES.

740 (protein) + 555 (fat) = 1,295 calories from protein and fat combined.

2,775 calories – 1,295 = 1,480 calories should come from carbs.

Again, remembering that there are FOUR calories in one gram of carbs, we divide this number by four to get into grams.

1,480/4 = 370 grams of carbs

-

Daily Calories: 2,775

Protein: 185 g

Fats: 62 g

Carbs: 370 g

-

Wasn't that fun?

Don't worry, you don't have to be Good Will Hunting smart (smot for you New Englanders) to be able to figure this out.

Like most things in life, there are APPS to make this way easier. MyFitnessPal is the one I use.

You can watch a video I made on how to set and track your calories and macros for effortless fat loss by searching 'Joel Staley Fitness Macros' on YouTube.

You like apples? How do you like dem apples?

Chapter 7: The Diet Trick That

WORKS

After finishing my first Men's Physique Show, you'll recall I mentioned going home and eating all the foods I had been craving for the last 12 weeks of sticking to my meal plan. The problem was, my stomach wasn't large enough to eat EVERYTHING I had been craving.

- Pizza.
- Nachos.
- Burgers.
- Brats.
- Donuts.
- Pancakes.
- Candy.
- Ice Cream.

The list went on and on.

This meant that I had to dedicate the next few days to eating all this junk. A few days came and went, and I quickly found that I couldn't control my eating. What I didn't know at the time was that binge eating was a common side effect from being on an insanely strict meal plan for too long, much like I had been for the 12 weeks leading up to my show. I told myself I had to stop with the junk, but even when I switched to eating healthy I knew I was consuming WAY too much food. I was eating big meals every 2-3 hours throughout the day!

This meant I had a huge breakfast at 5 am.

I was hungry again by 8 am, so I would eat again.

Hungry again by 11 am, eat again.

Hungry again by 2 pm, eat again.

Hungry again by 5 pm, eat again.

Hungry again by 7 pm, eat again.

Hungry again by 9 pm, eat again.

-

So one day, I decided to track my calories.

At the end of the day, after logging everything I had put in my mouth, I was at a whopping 5,700 calories!

I couldn't believe it. I was eating meat, vegetables, fruit, oatmeal, sweet potatoes, all of these "clean foods" and still WAY above my calories. My maintenance calories were around 2,700 at the time (meaning anything above that, I would gain weight) so I joked to my wife that I could LITERALLY NOT EAT the whole next day, and I'd still be over my calories for the two days combined!

Even though I said this as a joke, it did strike up a weird curiosity in me.

Do people fast?

Is fasting unhealthy?

Does it burn muscle?

The next day while I was eating breakfast before work, I decided to look up some videos in an effort to learn more about fasting. After watching my normal morning Ted Talk, I stumbled across a guy named Greg O'Gallagher preaching the awesomeness of something called Intermittent Fasting.

The basis was that he would only eat within an 8-hour window every day and then fast (or not eat) the remaining 16 hours of the day.

For example:

- Wake up at 7 am
- Fast until noon by only drinking black coffee and water
- Eat all your meals between noon and 8 pm.

- Then stop eating until noon the following day.

I decided that I would give it a try the following day and I have to say, I was impressed.

I went from uncontrollable binge eating to now having complete control over my hunger and the foods I put in my mouth. It doesn't make much sense at first. How did deciding I was only going to eat within this shorter window help these constant hunger pangs I was having?

What I found out was; I was eating breakfast first thing in the morning out of habit, before I was even hungry. This would cause my blood sugar and insulin levels to rise, which is fine, until about 2-3 hours later when they would start coming back down. This would send the signal to my brain that my levels are dipping, and I needed to eat something and QUICK! This process repeated itself every two to three hours throughout my day, causing me to constantly feel hungry. By pushing back my first meal until I was ACTUALLY hungry, much later in the day, I was able to save myself about eight hours of this agony.

After a few days of tracking, I saw I was around 2,000 calories a day, damn near cutting my calorie intake into thirds. I found that waking up and drinking a gallon of water before my first meal also helped suppress my appetite. After doing this for a few months and seeing all the benefits that fasting provided me, I decided to dive a little bit deeper and see what other types of fasting methods were out there.

Here are the five most common types of fasting that I've personally tried at some point to help me lose fat FAST (get it?), in order of my most favorite to least favorite.

-

1) Leangains Fasting - Typically fast for 16 hours and have an 8-hour eating window.

This was the first method of fasting I tried and had great success with. I would typically only drink water and black coffee until around 1 pm, then eat two or three meals between then and 9 pm. This helped me control my binge eating to the point that it went away rather quickly. I also felt great in the morning, like I had extra energy and focus. But maybe that was just all the coffee!

-

2) Prolonged Fasting - Fast for 24-72 hours (or longer).

Believe it or not, once you've mastered the Leangains approach, going 24 hours without food is a walk in the park. They do it on *Naked and Afraid* all the time, don't they? Not to mention the hundreds of thousands of years our hunter gatherer ancestors did it. So, you can make it a day, I promise.

The longest fast I've done to date was about 60 hours (or two and a half days). Knowing that I burn around 2,700 calories a day, that means I burned around 6,750 calories during that time without consuming any calories at all. If I were to diet at a 500 calorie deficit, **it would take me over 13 days to burn that much fat!** When it's broken down like that, you can see why fasting can make fat loss pretty damn easy.

I used this method of fasting after coming back from a three day bachelor party in Phoenix last year. I was only a month out from a Men's Physique Show and thought I was going to have to cancel because of this trip. I came back home to Nebraska and fasted for 36 hours, three separate times within two weeks. This is fairly aggressive and is not a recommendation, but I had a deadline to meet.

After the two weeks, not only had I undone all the damage I did in Arizona, I was looking better than I ever had before in my entire life! I ended up winning that fitness show and going pro, even though the competitors backstage were all talking about how they hadn't had a drink in months. As they were all talking about what their first drink was going to be, I couldn't help but think about the 40+ beers I had chugged in Phoenix just a few weeks prior.

-

3) Alternate Day Fasting

There are a couple different methods to this one. One method is done by eating regularly every other day and eating 1/5th of your normal calories every other day. For example, if your maintenance calories are 2,500 you would eat 2,500 calories Mon/Wed/Fri/Sun and eat 500 calories Tues/Thurs/Sat. The other method is to COMPLETELY fast every other 24 hours.

This method may be good for quick fat loss but probably isn't sustainable for most. I gave it a try for a couple weeks, but it was a little much for me.

-

4) Warrior Diet - This is when you fast all day and then eat one EPIC meal for dinner.

Some refer to this as the OMAD diet (or One Meal A Day diet).

This may be good for business professionals who have hectic work days and can't find the time to eat anything healthy while in and out of meetings all day. I tried this for a few months after leangains, but found it difficult to stick to it long term. If you decide to try it, you'll want to make sure you're getting enough protein to preserve your muscle, which can be hard to do in just one sitting.

-

5) Spontaneous Meal Skipping

Just like the name implies, this one is a bit less structured than the others. An example would be going on a business trip and not having any healthy options at the airport. If your choices are McDonalds or skipping a meal, you'd be better off skipping if your goal is fat loss. I do like using this method while flying to another city since there's hardly ever anything good to eat, the lines are long, and the food is expensive. If you're in a position like this and you're trying to lose some fat, instead of asking "What should I eat right now?" you can ask yourself, "Do I need to eat right now?".

-

Besides just fat loss, there are a ton of health benefits to fasting. Some studies now show that fasting preserves lean muscle mass better than just restricting calories. This is probably because naturally produced Human Growth Hormone (HGH) spikes dramatically while somebody is in a fasted state, sometimes upwards of 2,000% its normal level. This causes our bodies to burn body fat for energy instead of turning to muscle for fuel.

Think of it like this...

Do you think our bodies are storing excess energy in the form of fat only to burn muscle when it needs fuel?

Of course not.

Also, you might assume that since cutting your calories too low slows down your metabolism, not eating for days on end would slow it down significantly.

Nope.

Eating a small number of calories each day may actually be worse for your metabolism than not eating at all. By consuming these calories, you're not allowing your body to benefit from the many hormonal changes that take place during a fast. You're also preventing your body from burning body fat because it now has to digest the calories that you just ate.

-

So even though fasting isn't necessary for fat loss, it has been a major factor in helping me reach my fitness goals while also living in a way I enjoy. It may do the same for you.

Chapter 8: How Much Cardio To Do and What Types

Cardio is a great way to shed excess body fat, especially when your calories are already set low and you've plateaued in your fat loss. That being said, it should be an afterthought in the grand scheme of things. There's no reason you can't achieve your goals through resistance training, diet, and consistency alone. If you like doing cardio, it certainly won't hurt and can definitely speed up the process.

-

But so many cardio options to pick from...

Which one will work best for losing that stubborn belly fat without compromising your hard-earned muscle?

To find out, let's go over the different types of cardio.

-

LISS - Low Intensity Steady State

- Fast-Paced Walking
- Jogging
- Elliptical
- Steady Cycling

-

HIIT - High Intensity Interval Training

- Walk and Sprint
- Jog and Sprint
- Running Stairs
- Circuit Training

-

NEAT - Non-Exercise Activity Thermogenesis

Things we do throughout the day that we don't pay much attention to

- Walking
- Fidgeting
- Scratching your head
- Checking your watch
- Sniffing your arm pit, etc.

(Yes, these all burn calories and count as cardio)

-

So which one should you do?

A lot of guys will say that HIIT is the best way to lose the fat without increasing your odds of burning any muscle.

The problem with HIIT is if you haven't ran since senior year of high school, it could dramatically increase your risk of injury by pulling a muscle.

If this is the boat you're in, I would recommend focusing on NEAT (going on walks with the family around the neighborhood, parking further away at the store, taking the stairs instead of the elevator, etc.)

If you're really hell bent on doing REAL cardio, my second suggestion would be cycling. Cycling is a low impact form of cardio that's sure to get your heart racing. Otherwise, consider joining a basketball or racquetball league to get some extra cardio in and make some new buddies in the process.

-

How Much Cardio Should You Do?

If you're a skinnier dad and your primary goal is bulking up and building muscle, you should do little to no cardio. Cardio burns calories, which is counterproductive to building muscle.

-

If you're looking to shed some fat, you should do cardio 1-3 times per week secondary to resistance training. Ten to twenty minutes per session should do the trick. If your diet is in check, there's no need to go crazy. Keep in mind that you should never do your cardio BEFORE your resistance training session. The cardio will hinder your performance while lifting, so save it for after. You'll burn more fat saving it for after weightlifting anyway.

-

You may be tempted to ramp up the cardio in the first few weeks of your routine. Since you'll be losing fat from the diet and exercise, but also gaining muscle from lifting weights, the number on the scale will move very little or not at all. Remember, this book isn't how to lose weight, per say, but how to lose fat and build muscle. Doing both of these things, although offsetting on the scale, will cause you to look awesome.

Still, it can be pretty discouraging when the scale stays stagnant. A lot of guys will decide to throw in the towel on weightlifting and focus all their efforts on cardio in order to make that scale start dropping. To avoid being in this position, take progress pictures or get a body fat test done at the beginning of your program. These will be much more accurate than the scale in the first few months of transforming your physique. Once you've built a base of muscle, after a few months the number on the scale will start dropping as you continue to lose fat. You just need to make it until then.

-

Don't Overthink Cardio.

If you like it, do some. Just don't prioritize it over resistance training.

If you don't like it, don't do it. You can build a great physique without it.

Chapter 9: Your Step by Step Blueprint.

☐ Decide how many days per week you can commit to going to the gym.

_____ Days per week.

☐ Use this number to come up with the type of split you'll do.

Full Body/Upper-Lower/Upper-Lower-Full/Push-Pull-Legs

☐ Set a date that you're going to hit the gym no matter what.

Date and time: _____

☐ Figure out who's going to be your accountability partner.

_____

☐ Join the Dads Who Lift FB Group.

https://www.facebook.com/groups/Dads.Who.Lift/

☐ Download the MyFitnessPal app (add me Joel393).

Your username: _____

☐ Calculate your calories and macros in MyFitnessPal.

☐ Take Your "Before" Picture. Put it somewhere that will keep you driven to keep going.

☐ Go grocery shopping and meal prep for the week.

☐ Track your calories for one week consistently.

☐ Finish Your First Full Week of Lifting, Meal Prepping, and Tracking.

☐ Finish Your Second Week of Lifting, Meal Prepping, and Tracking.

☐ Finish Your Third Week of Lifting, Meal Prepping, and Tracking.

☐ Finish Your First Full Month of Lifting, Meal Prepping, and Tracking. Take Progress Picture.

☐ Finish Your Second Full Month of Lifting, Meal Prepping, and Tracking. Take Progress Picture.

☐ Finish Your Third Full Month of Lifting, Meal Prepping, and Tracking. Take Progress Picture.

Thanks for Reading!

Now that you have the answers you've been looking for, there's no reason you can't put them into action today.

If you've made it this far, I have no doubt that you're committed enough to build that lean, muscular physique you're after.

Need help setting up your training or nutrition plan?

Feel free to shoot me an email at joel@joelstaleyfitness.com and I'd be happy to help you out.

Made in the USA
Coppell, TX
14 June 2021